AUTOIMMUNE PALEO COOKBOOK

Dr. Kimberly Carlos

Copyright © 2023 by Dr. Kimberly Carlos

TABLE OF CONTENT

INTRODUCTION

Sarah had always been an active and vibrant woman, until an unexpected diagnosis shook her world. Her doctors confirmed that she had an autoimmune disease that left her exhausted, in constant pain, and struggling to enjoy even the simplest of pleasures. Determined to regain her health and vitality, she turned to the Autoimmune Paleo (AIP) diet.

With unwavering determination, Sarah began her AIP journey. The diet involved eliminating inflammatory foods like grains, dairy, and nightshades while focusing on nutrient-rich alternatives. Her kitchen became a sanctuary for wholesome ingredients like fresh vegetables, lean proteins, and nourishing bone broths.

The first few weeks were a challenge. Sarah missed her favorite comfort foods, but her desire to heal propelled her forward. Gradually, her energy levels began to improve. The debilitating joint pain that had plagued her for years started to diminish.

Sarah's newfound energy allowed her to reconnect with her love for the outdoors. She started taking leisurely walks in the park, gradually progressing to more strenuous hikes. She even signed up for a yoga class, which had always seemed impossible during her worst days.

Over time, Sarah's perseverance paid off. Her autoimmune symptoms became less frequent and less severe. Her skin glowed with health, and she felt more alive than she had in years.

One day, Sarah's doctor marveled at her progress. He was amazed by her transformation and said her commitment to the AIP diet had likely played a significant role in her recovery. Sarah knew that she would have to stick to the AIP diet for the rest of her life, but it was a small price to pay for the return of her vitality.

As Sarah continued her journey, she became an advocate for the AIP diet, helping others find hope and healing just as she had. She knew that her story was a testament to the power of determination and the incredible ability of the body to heal when given the right nourishment.

CHAPTER ONE

How to Follow an Auto Immune Paleo Diet and its Benefits

Following an Autoimmune Paleo (AIP) diet can be challenging, but it can also offer significant benefits for individuals with autoimmune diseases by reducing inflammation and promoting healing.

Here's a step-by-step guide on how to follow an AIP diet effectively to maximize its benefits:

1. Educate Yourself: Start by thoroughly understanding the AIP diet and why it works. Learn about the foods to include and exclude, and how they impact autoimmune conditions. Knowledge is your strongest tool in maintaining compliance and seeing results.

2. Consult a Healthcare Professional: Before making any dietary changes, consult with a healthcare provider or a registered dietitian, especially if you have specific medical conditions. They can help tailor the diet to your individual needs and monitor your progress.

3. Elimination Phase:

- Remove Trigger Foods: Eliminate all potential trigger foods that are known to exacerbate autoimmune symptoms. These typically include grains, dairy, legumes, nightshades, eggs, nuts, seeds, and processed foods.
- Focus on Nutrient-Rich Foods: Emphasize nutrient-dense foods such as lean meats (grass-fed and pasture-raised if possible), fatty fish, a variety of non-starchy vegetables, and healthy fats like avocado and olive oil.

4. Meal Planning:

- Plan Your Meals: Plan your meals in advance to ensure you have AIP-compliant options readily available. Batch cooking can save time and make it easier to stick to the diet.
- Explore AIP Recipes: There are many AIP-friendly recipes available online that can add variety to your meals.

5. Gradual Reintroduction: After a period of strict elimination (usually a few weeks to a few months), some individuals may reintroduce certain foods one at a time to see how their body reacts.

This is a personalized process and should be done under the guidance of a healthcare professional.

6. Monitor Your Progress:

- Keep a food diary to track your meals, symptoms, and any changes you observe. This will help identify trigger foods and monitor improvements.
- Pay attention to how you feel both physically and mentally. Many people on the AIP diet report improved energy levels, reduced pain, and enhanced mental clarity.

7. Lifestyle Factors:

- Stress Management: Incorporate stress-reduction techniques such as yoga, meditation, or deep breathing exercises, as stress can worsen autoimmune symptoms.
- Adequate Sleep: Prioritize good sleep hygiene to support your body's healing processes.

8. Stay Hydrated: Drink plenty of water to maintain hydration and aid in digestion.

9. Supplements: Consider supplements under the guidance of a healthcare provider. Common supplements include vitamin D, omega-3 fatty acids, and probiotics.

10. Community and Support: Connect with others who are following the AIP diet, either through online forums, social media groups, or local support groups. Sharing experiences and tips can be motivating and helpful.

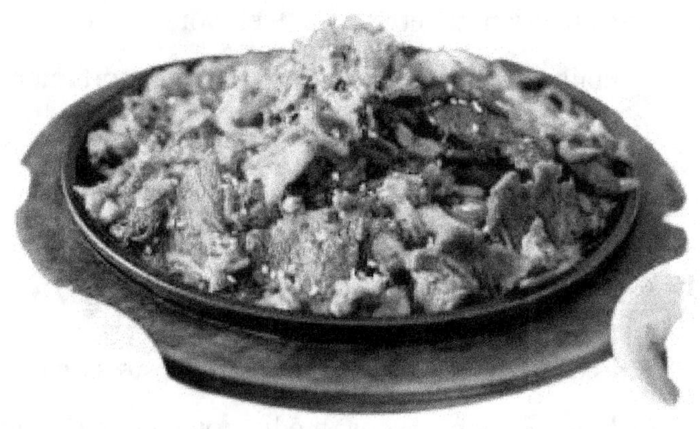

CHAPTER TWO

14-Day Autoimmune Paleo (AIP) Meal Plan

Day 1:

- Breakfast: Turkey and butternut squash hash with spinach.
- Lunch: Chicken and vegetable soup with bone broth.
- Dinner: Baked salmon with roasted broccoli and cauliflower.

Day 2:

- Breakfast: Avocado and bacon stuffed sweet potato.
- Lunch: A salad with mixed greens, shredded carrots, and shredded chicken, dressed with AIP-compliant dressing.
- Dinner: Grass-fed beef stew with carrots, parsnips, and onions.

Day 3:

- Breakfast: Blueberry and banana smoothie (using coconut milk and AIP-approved protein powder).
- Lunch: Turkey lettuce wraps with homemade guacamole.

- Dinner: Garlic and herb roasted chicken with sautéed asparagus.

Day 4:

- Breakfast: Beef and vegetable breakfast skillet.
- Lunch: Creamy butternut squash soup.
- Dinner: Lemon herb baked cod with sautéed kale.

Day 5:

- Breakfast: AIP-compliant sausage patties with mixed berries.
- Lunch: Turkey and vegetable stir-fry with coconut aminos.
- Dinner: Pork chops with applesauce and roasted Brussels sprouts.

Day 6:

- Breakfast: Sweet potato and sausage breakfast casserole.
- Lunch: Mixed greens salad with shredded turkey and balsamic vinaigrette.
- Dinner: Garlic and rosemary roasted lamb with mashed cauliflower.

Day 7:

- Breakfast: Zucchini and bacon fritters with avocado.
- Lunch: Chicken and vegetable curry (using coconut milk).
- Dinner: Baked cod with lemon and thyme, served with sautéed spinach.

Day 8:

- Breakfast: Apple and cinnamon porridge (made with grated apples and coconut).
- Lunch: Beef and vegetable soup with bone broth.
- Dinner: Turkey meatballs with AIP-compliant tomato sauce and zucchini noodles.

Day 9:

- Breakfast: Mixed berry smoothie (using coconut milk and AIP-approved protein powder).
- Lunch: A salad with mixed greens, shredded carrots, and shredded chicken, dressed with AIP-compliant dressing.
- Dinner: Grass-fed beef stir-fry with broccoli and cauliflower rice.

Day 10:

- Breakfast: Turkey and vegetable breakfast skillet.

- Lunch: Creamy butternut squash soup.

- Dinner: Lemon herb baked cod with sautéed kale.

Day 11:

- Breakfast: AIP-compliant sausage patties with mixed berries.

- Lunch: Turkey lettuce wraps with homemade guacamole.

- Dinner: Garlic and rosemary roasted lamb with mashed cauliflower.

Day 12:

- Breakfast: Sweet potato and sausage breakfast casserole.

- Lunch: Mixed greens salad with shredded turkey and balsamic vinaigrette.

- Dinner: Pork chops with applesauce and roasted Brussels sprouts.

Day 13:

- Breakfast: Zucchini and bacon fritters with avocado.
- Lunch: Chicken and vegetable curry (using coconut milk).
- Dinner: Baked salmon with roasted broccoli and cauliflower.

Day 14:

- Breakfast: Apple and cinnamon porridge (made with grated apples and coconut).
- Lunch: Beef and vegetable soup with bone broth.
- Dinner: Turkey meatballs with AIP-compliant tomato sauce and zucchini noodles.

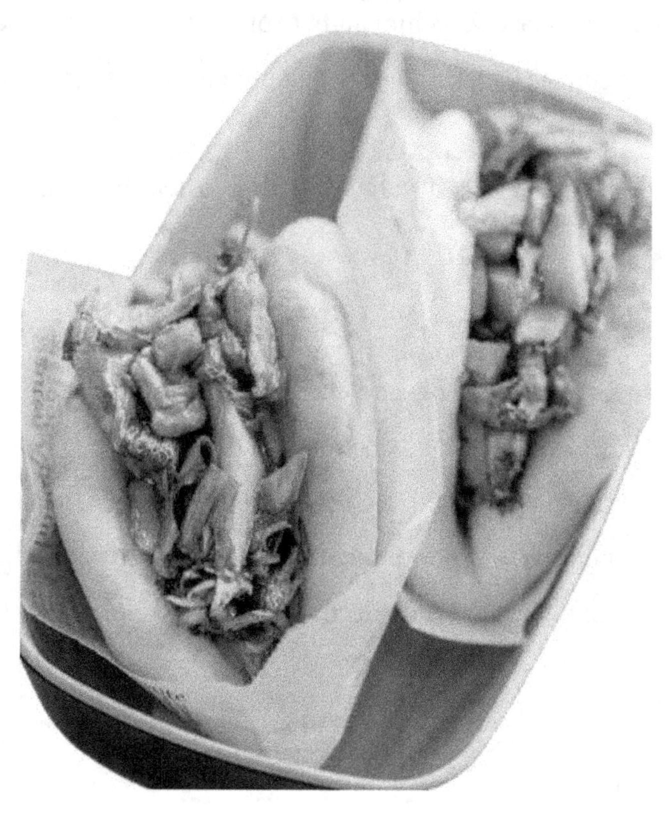

CHAPTER THREE

Auto Immune Paleo Breakfast Recipes

1. Sweet Potato Hash

A satisfying and hearty breakfast option that's AIP-compliant and packed with nutrients.

Ingredients:

- 2 medium sweet potatoes, peeled and grated
- 1 onion, diced
- 1/2 pound ground turkey
- 1 teaspoon turmeric
- Salt and pepper (omit pepper for AIP)
- Cooking fat (coconut oil or olive oil)

Instructions:

1. Heat cooking fat in a skillet over medium heat.

2. Add diced onion and cook until translucent.

3. Add ground turkey and cook until browned.

4. Add grated sweet potatoes, turmeric, salt, and pepper.

5. Cook for about 15-20 minutes, stirring occasionally, until

sweet potatoes are tender and slightly crispy.

6. Serve hot.

Cooking Time: 30-40 minutes

2. AIP Breakfast Sausage

Homemade AIP sausage patties that are flavorful and free from additives.

Ingredients:

- 1 pound ground pork or turkey
- 1 teaspoon dried sage
- 1/2 teaspoon dried thyme
- 1/2 teaspoon garlic powder
- 1/4 teaspoon salt
- 1/4 teaspoon black pepper (omit for AIP)
- Cooking fat (coconut oil or olive oil)

Instructions:

1. In a bowl, combine ground meat with sage, thyme, garlic powder, salt, and pepper.

2. Form the mixture into small patties.

3. Heat cooking fat in a skillet over medium-high heat.

4. Cook the patties for about 3-4 minutes on each side until they are cooked through.

5. Serve hot.

Cooking Time: 15-20 minutes

3. AIP Breakfast Smoothie

A nutritious and easy-to-make AIP-compliant breakfast option.

Ingredients:

- 1 ripe banana
- 1/2 cup diced cooked sweet potato
- 1/2 cup coconut milk
- 1/2 cup water
- 1 tablespoon honey (optional, omit for strict AIP)
- 1/2 teaspoon cinnamon

Instructions:

1. Place all ingredients in a blender.

2. Blend until smooth.

3. Adjust the thickness by adding more water if necessary.

4. Serve chilled.

Cooking Time: 5 minutes

4. Bacon-Wrapped Asparagus

A simple but elegant breakfast side dish that's AIP-friendly.

Ingredients:

-   12 asparagus spears
-   6 slices of AIP-compliant bacon

Instructions:

1. Preheat your oven to 375°F (190°C).

2. Wrap each asparagus spear with half a slice of bacon.

3. Place the wrapped asparagus on a baking sheet.

4. Bake for 15-20 minutes or until the bacon is crispy.

5. Serve hot.

Cooking Time: 20-25 minutes

5. Berry and Coconut Parfait

A refreshing and fruity AIP breakfast parfait.

Ingredients:

- 1 cup mixed berries (blueberries, strawberries, raspberries)
- 1 cup coconut yogurt (AIP-compliant)
- 1/4 cup shredded coconut
- 1 tablespoon honey (optional, omit for strict AIP)

Instructions:

1. In a glass or bowl, layer coconut yogurt, mixed berries, and shredded coconut.

2. Drizzle with honey if desired.

3. Repeat the layers.

4. Serve chilled.

Cooking Time: 5 minutes

6. Plantain Pancakes

Fluffy and naturally sweet AIP pancakes made from ripe plantains.

Ingredients:

- 2 ripe plantains
- 2 tablespoons coconut flour
- 1/4 cup coconut milk
- 1/2 teaspoon baking soda
- 1/4 teaspoon cinnamon
- Cooking fat (coconut oil or olive oil)

Instructions:

1. Peel and chop the ripe plantains.

2. Place plantains, coconut flour, coconut milk, baking soda, and cinnamon in a blender.

3. Blend until smooth.

4. Heat cooking fat in a skillet over medium heat.

5. Pour pancake batter onto the skillet to form pancakes.

6. Cook for 2-3 minutes on each side until golden brown.

7. Serve hot.

Cooking Time: 15-20 minutes

7. AIP Breakfast Casserole

A hearty and filling AIP breakfast casserole that's perfect for meal prep.

Ingredients:

- 1 pound ground beef or turkey
- 1 onion, diced
- 2 cups diced sweet potatoes
- 2 cups spinach
- 6-8 large eggs (or AIP-compliant egg substitute)
- Salt and pepper (omit pepper for AIP)
- Cooking fat (coconut oil or olive oil)

Instructions:

1. Preheat your oven to 375°F (190°C).

2. In a skillet, cook ground meat and onion until browned.

3. In a separate skillet, sauté sweet potatoes until they begin to soften.

4. In a greased baking dish, layer cooked sweet potatoes,

spinach, and the meat mixture.

5. In a bowl, whisk eggs with salt and pepper (if using).

6. Pour the egg mixture over the layers.

7. Bake for 25-30 minutes or until the eggs are set.

8. Serve hot or refrigerate for later use.

Cooking Time: 45-60 minutes

8. Avocado and Bacon Stuffed Sweet Potato

A creamy and savory AIP breakfast that's both satisfying and nutritious.

Ingredients:

- 2 sweet potatoes
- 1 avocado
- 4 slices AIP-compliant bacon, cooked and crumbled
- Chopped fresh parsley (for garnish)
- Salt and pepper (omit pepper for AIP)

Instructions:

1. Preheat your oven to 375°F (190°C).

2. Bake sweet potatoes for 45-60 minutes until tender.

3. Cut each sweet potato in half and scoop out some of the flesh to create a hollow.

4. Mash the scooped-out sweet potato flesh with avocado, bacon, salt, and pepper.

5. Stuff the sweet potato halves with the avocado-bacon mixture.

6. Garnish with chopped parsley.

7. Serve hot.

Cooking Time: 60-75 minutes

9. AIP Breakfast Soup

A warm and comforting AIP breakfast option that's packed with nutrients.

Ingredients:

-   2 cups bone broth (AIP-compliant)

- 1 cup diced cooked chicken
- 1 cup chopped mixed vegetables (carrots, celery, zucchini)
- 1/2 teaspoon dried thyme
- Salt and pepper (omit pepper for AIP)

Instructions:

1. In a pot, combine bone broth, chicken, mixed vegetables, thyme, salt, and pepper (if using).

2. Bring to a simmer and cook for 10-15 minutes until vegetables are tender.

3. Serve hot.

Cooking Time: 20-30 minutes

10. Coconut and Banana Porridge

A warm and comforting AIP porridge that's reminiscent of traditional oatmeal.

Ingredients:

- 2 ripe bananas
- 1/2 cup shredded coconut

- 1/2 cup coconut milk

- 1/2 teaspoon cinnamon

- 1/4 teaspoon vanilla extract (omit for strict AIP)

Instructions:

1. In a blender, combine ripe bananas, shredded coconut, coconut milk, cinnamon, and vanilla extract (if using).

2. Blend until smooth.

3. Pour the mixture into a saucepan and heat over medium heat until it thickens, stirring constantly.

4. Serve warm.

Cooking Time: 10-15 minutes

Auto Immune Paleo Lunch Recipes

1. AIP Chicken Salad

A refreshing and nutrient-packed AIP chicken salad with a creamy dressing.

Ingredients:

- 2 cups shredded cooked chicken
- 1/2 cup diced cucumber
- 1/2 cup diced celery
- 1/4 cup chopped fresh parsley
- 1/4 cup AIP-compliant mayo (homemade or store-bought)
- 1 tablespoon apple cider vinegar
- Salt and pepper (omit pepper for AIP)

Instructions:

1. In a large bowl, combine shredded chicken, cucumber, celery, and fresh parsley.

2. In a separate bowl, whisk together AIP-compliant mayo, apple cider vinegar, salt, and pepper (if using).

3. Pour the dressing over the chicken mixture and toss until

well coated.

4. Chill before serving.

Cooking Time: 10-15 minutes

2. AIP Turkey and Sweet Potato Hash

A savory and hearty AIP hash with the sweetness of sweet potatoes.

Ingredients:

- 1 pound ground turkey
- 2 cups diced sweet potatoes
- 1/2 cup diced onion
- 1/2 cup diced bell peppers
- 1/4 cup chopped fresh cilantro
- Cooking fat (coconut oil or olive oil)
- Salt and pepper (omit pepper for AIP)

Instructions:

1. Heat cooking fat in a skillet over medium-high heat.

2. Add ground turkey and cook until browned.

3. Remove turkey from the skillet and set aside.

4. In the same skillet, add more cooking fat if needed, then add sweet potatoes, onion, and bell peppers.

5. Cook until sweet potatoes are tender and slightly crispy.

6. Return the cooked turkey to the skillet, add fresh cilantro, and season with salt and pepper (if using).

7. Cook for a few more minutes, stirring to combine.

8. Serve hot.

Cooking Time: 30-40 minutes

3. AIP Tuna Salad

A quick and easy AIP tuna salad with a zesty dressing.

Ingredients:

- 2 cans of AIP-compliant tuna, drained
- 1/2 cup diced cucumber
- 1/2 cup diced celery
- 1/4 cup chopped fresh dill
- Juice of 1 lemon
- 2 tablespoons olive oil
- Salt and pepper (omit pepper for AIP)

Instructions:

1. In a large bowl, combine drained tuna, cucumber, celery, and fresh dill.

2. In a small bowl, whisk together lemon juice, olive oil, salt, and pepper (if using).

3. Pour the dressing over the tuna mixture and toss until well combined.

4. Chill before serving.

Cooking Time: 10 minutes

4. AIP Beef and Broccoli Stir-Fry

A tasty and nutrient-dense AIP stir-fry with tender beef and crisp broccoli.

Ingredients:

- 1 pound thinly sliced beef
- 2 cups broccoli florets
- 1/2 cup sliced carrots
- 1/4 cup coconut aminos
- 2 cloves garlic, minced

- 1 teaspoon grated ginger

- Cooking fat (coconut oil or olive oil)

- Salt and pepper (omit pepper for AIP)

Instructions:

1. Heat cooking fat in a skillet or wok over high heat.

2. Add sliced beef and cook until browned.

3. Remove beef from the skillet and set aside.

4. In the same skillet, add more cooking fat if needed, then add broccoli, carrots, garlic, and ginger.

5. Stir-fry until vegetables are tender.

6. Return the cooked beef to the skillet, add coconut aminos, and season with salt and pepper (if using).

7. Cook for a few more minutes, stirring to combine.

8. Serve hot.

Cooking Time: 20-25 minutes

5. AIP Zucchini Noodles with Pesto

A light and flavorful AIP lunch with zucchini noodles and a basil pesto sauce.

Ingredients:

- 2 medium zucchinis, spiralized into noodles
- 1 cup fresh basil leaves
- 1/4 cup olive oil
- 2 cloves garlic, minced
- Juice of 1 lemon
- Salt (omit pepper for AIP)

Instructions:

1. In a blender or food processor, combine fresh basil, olive oil, garlic, lemon juice, and salt.

2. Blend until smooth to make the pesto sauce.

3. In a skillet, sauté the zucchini noodles over medium heat until they're tender.

4. Toss the zucchini noodles with the pesto sauce.

5. Serve warm or cold.

Cooking Time: 15-20 minutes

6. AIP Chicken and Vegetable Soup

A comforting and nourishing AIP soup filled with chicken and veggies.

Ingredients:

- 2 cups shredded cooked chicken
- 4 cups AIP-compliant chicken broth
- 2 cups mixed vegetables (carrots, celery, squash)
- 1/2 cup chopped fresh parsley
- Salt and pepper (omit pepper for AIP)

Instructions:

1. In a pot, combine shredded chicken, chicken broth, mixed vegetables, and fresh parsley.

2. Bring to a simmer and cook until the vegetables are tender.

3. Season with salt and pepper (if using).

4. Serve hot.

Cooking Time: 20-30 minutes

7. AIP Salmon Salad

A light and refreshing AIP salad with poached salmon.

Ingredients:

- 2 salmon fillets
- 4 cups mixed greens
- 1/2 cucumber, sliced
- 1/2 cup sliced radishes
- 1/4 cup chopped fresh dill
- Juice of 1 lemon
- 2 tablespoons olive oil
- Salt and pepper (omit pepper for AIP)

Instructions:

1. Poach the salmon fillets by gently simmering in water for about 10 minutes until cooked through.

2. In a large bowl, combine mixed greens, sliced cucumber, sliced radishes, and fresh dill.

3. In a small bowl, whisk together lemon juice, olive oil, salt, and pepper (if using).

4. Drizzle the dressing over the salad and toss to combine.

5. Place poached salmon fillets on top.

6. Serve chilled.

Cooking Time: 15-20 minutes

8. AIP Turkey Lettuce Wraps

A light and crunchy AIP lunch option using lettuce leaves as wraps.

Ingredients:

- 1 pound ground turkey
- 1/2 cup diced bell peppers
- 1/2 cup diced cucumber
- 1/4 cup chopped fresh mint leaves
- Juice of 1 lime
- Salt and pepper (omit pepper for AIP)
- Large lettuce leaves (such as iceberg or butter lettuce)

Instructions:

1. In a skillet, cook ground turkey until browned.

2. In a bowl, combine cooked turkey, diced bell peppers,

diced cucumber, fresh mint, lime juice, salt, and pepper (if using).

3. Spoon the turkey mixture into lettuce leaves to create wraps.

4. Serve cold.

Cooking Time: 15-20 minutes

9. AIP Roasted Vegetable Salad

A colorful and hearty AIP salad featuring roasted vegetables.

Ingredients:

- 2 cups mixed greens
- 1 cup roasted sweet potatoes
- 1 cup roasted beets
- 1/2 cup sliced red onion
- 1/4 cup chopped fresh parsley
- AIP-compliant dressing of your choice

Instructions:

1. Toss mixed greens, roasted sweet potatoes, roasted beets, sliced red onion, and fresh parsley in a large bowl.

2. Drizzle with your favorite AIP-compliant dressing.

3. Serve cold or at room temperature.

Cooking Time: 30-40 minutes (for roasting)

10. AIP Cauliflower Fried Rice

A satisfying AIP-friendly fried "rice" made with cauliflower.

Ingredients:

- 1 head cauliflower, grated into rice-sized pieces
- 1 cup diced cooked chicken
- 1/2 cup diced carrots
- 1/2 cup diced zucchini
- 1/4 cup chopped green onions (green parts only)
- 2 tablespoons coconut aminos
- Cooking fat (coconut oil or olive oil)
- Salt and pepper (omit pepper for AIP)

Instructions:

1. Heat cooking fat in a large skillet or wok over medium-high heat.

2. Add grated cauliflower and cook until it starts to brown slightly.

3. Add diced chicken, diced carrots, and diced zucchini.

4. Cook until the vegetables are tender.

5. Stir in chopped green onions and coconut aminos.

6. Season with salt and pepper (if using).

7. Cook for a few more minutes, stirring to combine.

8. Serve hot.

Cooking Time: 20-25 minutes

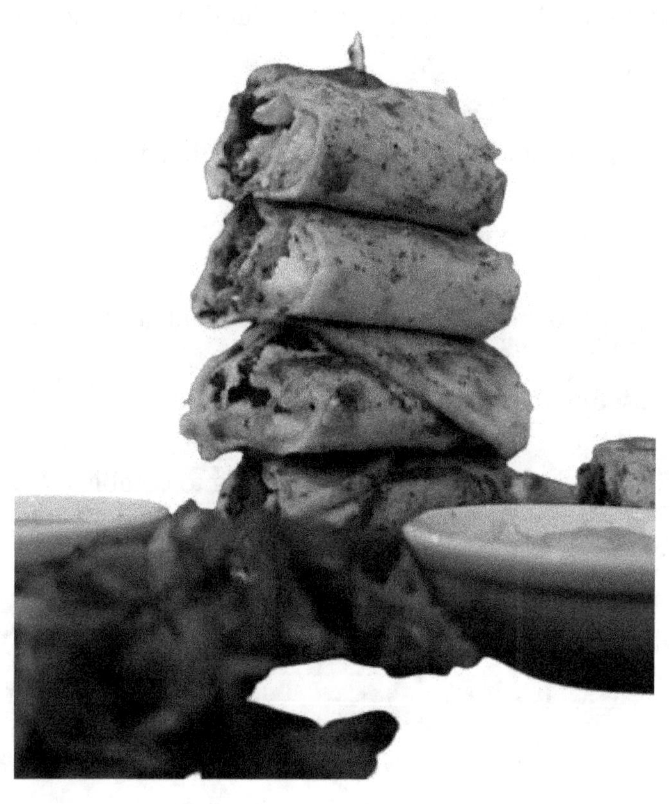

CHAPTER FOUR

Auto Immune Paleo Dinner Recipes

1. AIP Baked Chicken Thighs

A simple and flavorful AIP dinner with juicy baked chicken thighs.

Ingredients:

- 4 bone-in, skin-on chicken thighs
- 1 tablespoon olive oil
- 1 teaspoon dried thyme
- 1 teaspoon garlic powder
- Salt and pepper (omit pepper for AIP)

Instructions:

1. Preheat your oven to 375°F (190°C).

2. Rub chicken thighs with olive oil and season with dried thyme, garlic powder, salt, and pepper (if using).

3. Place chicken thighs on a baking sheet.

4. Bake for 35-40 minutes or until the chicken is cooked through and juices run clear.

5. Serve hot.

Cooking Time: 40-45 minutes

2. AIP Spaghetti Squash with Meat Sauce

A comforting AIP dinner with spaghetti squash and a flavorful meat sauce.

Ingredients:

- 1 spaghetti squash
- 1 pound ground beef
- 1 onion, diced
- 2 cloves garlic, minced
- 2 cups AIP-compliant tomato sauce
- 1 teaspoon dried basil
- Salt and pepper (omit pepper for AIP)

Instructions:

1. Preheat your oven to 375°F (190°C).

2. Cut the spaghetti squash in half lengthwise and scoop out the seeds.

3. Place the squash halves, cut side down, on a baking sheet.

4. Bake for 30-40 minutes or until the squash flesh is tender

and shreds easily with a fork.

5. While the squash is baking, in a skillet, cook ground beef, diced onion, and minced garlic until browned.

6. Stir in AIP-compliant tomato sauce and dried basil.

7. Season with salt and pepper (if using).

8. Simmer for 10-15 minutes.

9. Once the squash is cooked, scrape the flesh with a fork to create spaghetti-like strands.

10. Serve the meat sauce over the spaghetti squash.

Cooking Time: 40-55 minutes

3. AIP Lemon Herb Roasted Salmon

A light and flavorful AIP dinner featuring oven-roasted salmon.

Ingredients:

- 4 salmon fillets
- Zest and juice of 1 lemon
- 2 tablespoons chopped fresh dill

-   1 tablespoon olive oil

-   Salt and pepper (omit pepper for AIP)

Instructions:

1. Preheat your oven to 375°F (190°C).

2. In a small bowl, combine lemon zest, lemon juice, fresh dill, olive oil, salt, and pepper (if using).

3. Place salmon fillets on a baking sheet.

4. Drizzle the lemon herb mixture over the salmon.

5. Bake for 15-20 minutes or until the salmon flakes easily with a fork.

6. Serve hot.

Cooking Time: 15-20 minutes

4. AIP Beef and Broccoli Stir-Fry

A savory and satisfying AIP stir-fry with tender beef and broccoli.

Ingredients:

- 1 pound thinly sliced beef
- 2 cups broccoli florets
- 1/2 cup sliced carrots
- 1/4 cup coconut aminos
- 2 cloves garlic, minced
- 1 teaspoon grated ginger
- Cooking fat (coconut oil or olive oil)
- Salt and pepper (omit pepper for AIP)

Instructions:

1. Heat cooking fat in a skillet or wok over high heat.

2. Add sliced beef and cook until browned.

3. Remove beef from the skillet and set aside.

4. In the same skillet, add more cooking fat if needed, then add broccoli, carrots, garlic, and ginger.

5. Stir-fry until vegetables are tender.

6. Return the cooked beef to the skillet, add coconut aminos, and season with salt and pepper (if using).

7. Cook for a few more minutes, stirring to combine.

8. Serve hot.

Cooking Time: 20-25 minutes

5. AIP Pork Chops with Applesauce

A comforting and sweet AIP dinner featuring tender pork chops and homemade applesauce.

Ingredients:

- 4 pork chops
- 4 apples, peeled, cored, and chopped
- 1/2 cup water
- 1/2 teaspoon cinnamon
- Salt and pepper (omit pepper for AIP)
- Cooking fat (coconut oil or olive oil)

Instructions:

1. In a skillet, heat cooking fat over medium-high heat.

2. Season pork chops with salt and pepper (if using).

3. Cook pork chops until browned on both sides and cooked through (about 5-7 minutes per side).

4. While the pork chops are cooking, in a separate pot, combine chopped apples, water, and cinnamon.

5. Simmer over medium heat until the apples are soft and can be easily mashed with a fork.

6. Mash the apples to create applesauce.

7. Serve the pork chops with a dollop of homemade applesauce.

Cooking Time: 20-25 minutes

6. AIP Garlic and Rosemary Roasted Lamb

A hearty and aromatic AIP dinner featuring tender roasted lamb.

- **Ingredients:**
- 2 pounds boneless lamb shoulder roast
- 4 cloves garlic, minced
- 2 tablespoons chopped fresh rosemary
- 2 tablespoons olive oil
- Salt and pepper (omit pepper for AIP)

Instructions:

1. Preheat your oven to 375°F (190°C).

2. In a small bowl, combine minced garlic, chopped fresh rosemary, olive oil, salt, and pepper (if using).

3. Rub the garlic and rosemary mixture over the lamb roast.

4. Place the lamb roast on a baking sheet.

5. Bake for 30-40 minutes or until the lamb reaches your desired level of doneness (medium-rare, medium, etc.).

6. Remove from the oven and let it rest for a few minutes before slicing.

7. Serve hot.

Cooking Time: 40-50 minutes

7. AIP Lemon and Herb Roasted Chicken

A classic and savory AIP dinner featuring whole roasted chicken with lemon and herbs.

Ingredients:

- 1 whole chicken (3-4 pounds)
- Zest and juice of 1 lemon
- 2 tablespoons chopped fresh herbs (such as rosemary, thyme, or oregano)
- 2 tablespoons olive oil
- Salt and pepper (omit pepper for AIP)

Instructions:

1. Preheat your oven to 375°F (190°C).

2. In a small bowl, combine lemon zest, lemon juice, chopped fresh herbs, olive oil, salt, and pepper (if using).

3. Place the whole chicken in a roasting pan.

4. Brush the lemon and herb mixture over the chicken.

5. Roast the chicken for 60-75 minutes or until the internal temperature reaches 165°F (74°C) and the skin is crispy.

6. Let the chicken rest for a few minutes before carving.

7. Serve hot.

Cooking Time: 60-75 minutes

8. AIP Cauliflower and Parsnip Mash

A creamy and comforting AIP side dish made from cauliflower and parsnips.

Ingredients:

- 1 head cauliflower, cut into florets
- 2 parsnips, peeled and chopped
- 2 tablespoons coconut oil
- 2 cloves garlic, minced
- Salt and pepper (omit pepper for AIP)

Instructions:

1. Steam cauliflower florets and chopped parsnips until they are very tender (about 15-20 minutes).

2. Drain the vegetables and transfer them to a food processor.

3. Add coconut oil, minced garlic, salt, and pepper (if using).

4. Process until the mixture is smooth and creamy.

5. Serve hot as a side dish.

Cooking Time: 15-20 minutes

9. AIP Cabbage and Ground Beef Skillet

A budget-friendly and flavorful AIP dinner featuring ground beef and sautéed cabbage.

Ingredients:

- 1 pound ground beef
- 1 small head cabbage, thinly sliced
- 1 onion, diced
- 2 cloves garlic, minced
- 2 tablespoons coconut oil
- Salt and pepper (omit pepper for AIP)

Instructions:

1. In a large skillet, heat coconut oil over medium-high heat.

2. Add diced onion and minced garlic and sauté until fragrant.

3. Add ground beef and cook until browned.

4. Stir in thinly sliced cabbage.

5. Cook, stirring occasionally, until the cabbage is tender.

6. Season with salt and pepper (if using).

7. Serve hot.

Cooking Time: 20-25 minutes

10. AIP Turkey Meatballs with Tomato Sauce

A tasty and satisfying AIP dinner with turkey meatballs and AIP-compliant tomato sauce.

Ingredients:

- 1 pound ground turkey
- 1/4 cup finely chopped onion
- 1/4 cup chopped fresh basil
- 1/4 cup chopped fresh parsley
- 2 cups AIP-compliant tomato sauce
- Salt and pepper (omit pepper for AIP)
- Cooking fat (coconut oil or olive oil)

Instructions:

1. Preheat your oven to 375°F (190°C).

2. In a bowl, combine ground turkey, chopped onion, chopped basil, chopped parsley, salt, and pepper (if using).

3. Form the mixture into small meatballs.

4. Heat cooking fat in a skillet over medium-high heat.

5. Brown the meatballs on all sides.

6. Transfer the meatballs to a baking dish and pour AIP-compliant tomato sauce over them.

7. Bake for 20-25 minutes or until the meatballs are cooked through.

8. Serve hot with extra sauce if desired.

Cooking Time: 40-50 minutes

Auto Immune Paleo Snacks Recipes

1. AIP Avocado and Bacon Bites

A simple and satisfying AIP snack combining creamy avocado with crispy bacon.

Ingredients:

- 2 ripe avocados
- 4 slices AIP-compliant bacon, cooked and crumbled
- Salt and pepper (omit pepper for AIP)

Instructions:

1. Cut the avocados in half, remove the pits, and scoop out some flesh to create a hollow.

2. Sprinkle the avocado halves with crumbled bacon.

3. Season with a pinch of salt and pepper (if using).

4. Serve immediately.

Preparation Time: 10 minutes

2. AIP Sweet Potato Chips

Crispy and flavorful sweet potato chips that make for a delicious AIP snack.

Ingredients:

- 2 large sweet potatoes, thinly sliced
- 2 tablespoons coconut oil
- Salt (omit pepper for AIP)

Instructions:

1. Preheat your oven to 300°F (150°C).

2. Toss sweet potato slices with melted coconut oil and a pinch of salt.

3. Arrange the slices in a single layer on a baking sheet.

4. Bake for 25-30 minutes, flipping the slices halfway through, until they are crisp.

5. Let cool before serving.

Preparation Time: 40-45 minutes

3. AIP Guacamole with Veggie Sticks

Classic guacamole paired with fresh vegetable sticks for a nutritious AIP snack.

Ingredients:

- 2 ripe avocados
- Juice of 1 lime
- 2 cloves garlic, minced
- 2 tablespoons chopped fresh cilantro
- Carrot sticks, cucumber slices, and celery sticks (for dipping)
- Salt and pepper (omit pepper for AIP)

Instructions:

1. In a bowl, mash the avocados.

2. Stir in lime juice, minced garlic, chopped cilantro, salt, and pepper (if using).

3. Serve the guacamole with carrot sticks, cucumber slices, and celery sticks for dipping.

Preparation Time: 15 minutes

4. AIP Beef Jerky

Homemade AIP beef jerky with simple seasonings for a protein-packed snack.

Ingredients:

- 1 pound lean beef, thinly sliced
- 1/4 cup coconut aminos
- 1/2 teaspoon garlic powder
- 1/2 teaspoon onion powder
- 1/4 teaspoon ground ginger
- Salt and pepper (omit pepper for AIP)

Instructions:

1. In a bowl, combine coconut aminos, garlic powder, onion powder, ground ginger, salt, and pepper (if using).

2. Marinate the thinly sliced beef in the mixture for at least 30 minutes.

3. Preheat your oven to the lowest setting (usually around 150-170°F or 65-75°C).

4. Place the marinated beef slices on a baking rack set over a baking sheet.

5. Bake for 4-6 hours until the beef is dried and jerky-like.

6. Let cool before storing.

Preparation Time: 4-6 hours (mostly inactive)

5. AIP Cucumber and Tuna Bites

A light and refreshing AIP snack featuring cucumber slices topped with tuna salad.

Ingredients:

-   1 cucumber, sliced into rounds
-   1 can of AIP-compliant tuna, drained
-   1/4 cup diced red onion
-   1/4 cup diced cucumber
-   1 tablespoon olive oil
-   1 tablespoon apple cider vinegar
-   Salt and pepper (omit pepper for AIP)

Instructions:

1. In a bowl, combine drained tuna, diced red onion, diced cucumber, olive oil, apple cider vinegar, salt, and pepper (if using).

2. Place a spoonful of the tuna salad on each cucumber slice.

3. Serve immediately.

Preparation Time: 15 minutes

6. AIP Veggie Roll-Ups

Crunchy and colorful veggie roll-ups filled with a tasty AIP dip.

Ingredients:

- 2 large carrots, peeled and thinly sliced into strips
- 2 large zucchinis, thinly sliced into strips
- 1/2 cup AIP-compliant guacamole or hummus (store-bought or homemade)
- Salt and pepper (omit pepper for AIP)

Instructions:

1. Lay a carrot strip and a zucchini strip side by side.

2. Spread a thin layer of AIP-compliant guacamole or hummus on the strips.

3. Roll the strips together.

4. Repeat with the remaining strips.

5. Season with a pinch of salt and pepper (if using).

6. Serve chilled.

Preparation Time: 15 minutes

7. AIP Artichoke and Olive Tapenade

A tangy and briny AIP dip served with veggie sticks or plantain chips.

Ingredients:

- 1 can of AIP-compliant artichoke hearts, drained and chopped
- 1/2 cup pitted green olives, chopped
- 2 tablespoons olive oil
- Juice of 1 lemon
- 2 cloves garlic, minced
- Salt and pepper (omit pepper for AIP)

Instructions:

1. In a bowl, combine chopped artichoke hearts, chopped green olives, olive oil, lemon juice, minced garlic, salt, and pepper (if using).

2. Mix well.

3. Serve with veggie sticks or plantain chips.

Preparation Time: 10 minutes

8. AIP Plantain Chips with Guacamole

Crispy AIP plantain chips paired with creamy guacamole for a satisfying snack.

Ingredients:

- 2 green plantains, peeled and thinly sliced
- 2 tablespoons coconut oil
- Salt (omit pepper for AIP)
- 2 ripe avocados
- Juice of 1 lime
- 2 cloves garlic, minced
- 2 tablespoons chopped fresh cilantro

Instructions:

1. Preheat your oven to 350°F (175°C).

2. Toss plantain slices with melted coconut oil and a pinch of salt.

3. Arrange the slices in a single layer on a baking sheet.

4. Bake for 15-20 minutes, flipping the slices halfway through, until they are crisp.

5. While the plantains are baking, prepare guacamole by mashing ripe avocados and mixing with lime juice, minced garlic, chopped cilantro, salt, and pepper (if using).

6. Serve the plantain chips with guacamole.

Preparation Time: 30-35 minutes

9. AIP Mixed Berry Parfait

A sweet and fruity AIP parfait made with mixed berries and coconut yogurt.

Ingredients:

- 1 cup mixed AIP-compliant berries (such as

strawberries, blueberries, and raspberries)

- 1 cup AIP-compliant coconut yogurt (store-bought or homemade)

- 2 tablespoons shredded coconut

Instructions:

1. In a glass or jar, layer mixed berries, coconut yogurt, and shredded coconut.

2. Repeat the layers as desired.

3. Serve chilled.

Preparation Time: 10 minutes

10. AIP Trail Mix

A homemade AIP trail mix packed with nuts, seeds, and dried fruit.

Ingredients:

- 1 cup mixed AIP-compliant nuts (such as almonds, cashews, and macadamia nuts)

- 1/2 cup unsweetened dried cherries or cranberries

- 1/4 cup toasted coconut flakes

- 2 tablespoons pumpkin seeds

- 2 tablespoons sunflower seeds

- 1/2 teaspoon ground cinnamon

- Pinch of salt (omit pepper for AIP)

Instructions:

1. In a bowl, combine mixed nuts, dried cherries or cranberries, toasted coconut flakes, pumpkin seeds, sunflower seeds, ground cinnamon, salt, and pepper (if using).

2. Mix well.

3. Store in an airtight container for a convenient on-the-go snack.

Preparation Time: 10 minutes

CONCLUSION

In conclusion, the Autoimmune Paleo (AIP) diet stands as a valuable and carefully crafted nutritional approach for individuals struggling with autoimmune conditions. This dietary regimen has gained significant attention and recognition for its potential to alleviate symptoms, reduce inflammation, and promote overall health. As we've explored in this overview, the AIP diet is built on a foundation of removing potential triggers and incorporating healing foods.

One of the core strengths of the AIP diet is its focus on eliminating foods that commonly contribute to inflammation and autoimmune reactions. By cutting out grains, dairy, legumes, processed foods, and certain spices, it aims to reduce the burden on the immune system and allow the body to heal.

Simultaneously, the AIP diet encourages the consumption of nutrient-dense, healing foods. These include a variety of fruits, vegetables, high-quality proteins, healthy fats, and herbs. These components provide essential vitamins, minerals, antioxidants, and phytonutrients that support the immune system, gut health, and overall well-being.

Furthermore, the AIP diet emphasizes the removal of potential gut irritants, as the gut plays a pivotal role in autoimmune conditions. By excluding foods like gluten, which can contribute to leaky gut, and incorporating gut-healing foods like bone broth, the AIP diet addresses the underlying mechanisms of autoimmunity.

While the AIP diet can be a powerful tool in managing autoimmune conditions, it's essential to approach it with care and under the guidance of a healthcare provider or registered dietitian. It may not be suitable for everyone, and individual dietary needs and responses can vary significantly.

In addition to its potential health benefits, the AIP diet has sparked innovation in the culinary world, leading to a wide range of creative and delicious recipes that cater to those with autoimmune conditions. This has allowed individuals to enjoy flavorful meals while adhering to the AIP guidelines.

With careful planning and a commitment to its principles, the AIP diet offers hope and healing for many on their journey to managing autoimmune conditions.

www.ingramcontent.com/pod-product-compliance
Lightning Source LLC
Chambersburg PA
CBHW050851260726

48660CB00006B/2576